Hello: I'm A Sugar Addict

How I managed to quit all added sugar for good and tools you can use to do the same.

Brian Maucere

DEDICATION

Aunt Eileen – This book would never have been written without you putting the bug in my ear years ago. Your support and love is greatly felt.

Pop – The smartest guy I know. At 38, I'm still trying to be more like you.

Sofia – What can I say? You were my inspiration to write this book and finally beat this addiction. You saved my life. I am so proud to be your daddy. I love you.

CONTENTS

ACKNOWLEDGMENTS

Writing this book has been a true joy and labor of love. In all, I wrote the first draft in less than three weeks. This reaffirms that it was the right thing to do and I am so glad you have chosen to read it. Yet, this book would not be possible without the unwavering love and affection of my wife, Amanda. Beyond being an outstanding dietitian and leader in nutrition, she is an amazing partner and friend. Having somebody in your corner can mean the difference between success and failure and it is not lost on me that I am lucky to have her in my life. My hope is this book inspires 1 person to take a deeper look at their own sugar addiction and make a change.

PART I

1 SUGAR MONSTERS

On June 2, 2012 my family was attending a high school graduation for one of our teen athletes. We were sitting in the far off bleachers because my daughter Sofia (who was a little over 2 at the time) loved to walk around and talk loudly. She was also doing a lot of word association at the time as she tried to put sentences together. She pointed at Amanda's water bottle and said, "Mommy?" Great, right? Well then she pointed at an empty Dr. Pepper bottle under the seats and said, "Daddy?" She had this big smile on her face as she looked up at me and I managed a "Good girl." Sofia went off playing, but I quietly stood there in the bleachers feeling crushed. I mean CRUSHED. Sofia was associating soda with me and water with my wife. I couldn't stop thinking about my sweet and smart little girl who was so proud of herself for making the connection. Over the next few days, she would repeat the words regardless if I was the one holding the soda or not. She would look up at us for confirmation and our approval and I would get more and more depressed. This was the first time Sofia encouraged me to make some changes. Within two weeks, I quit drinking soda.

I figured the only way to do it was to go cold turkey and stop drinking it. No big plan in place. No weening myself off. I would simply quit. I wasn't going to try and keep drinking it while hiding it from Sofia either. To help me get started, I figured out how much I was spending annually buying my Diet Dr. Peppers. It turned out to be almost the same as the annual Disney passes for the family. No joke. I was buying at least two 16 oz soda bottles a day at an average of $1.50 each. At $3 a day, I was shocked to find I spent over $1000 a year drinking soda. Annual passes at $900 ended up saving us money. I told Amanda my plan and she lovingly supported my decision.

I started the next week off strong. Since I usually bought a 16 oz soda when I stopped for gas, I made sure I had a full tank and only paid at the pump. That worked for about 2 days. Then the cravings kicked in. By Thursday I was a wreck. I hate to admit this, but I was pacing around my house trying to decide whether I was going to go get one soda from the convenience store so the cravings would stop. Somehow, I vetoed that idea and headed off to the grocery store instead. With zero plan in place, I walked up and down the aisles looking for a solution. Like some sort of cosmic test of my strength, I had to walk past a guy who was pouring out samples of a new soda flavor at the end of one of the aisles. Seriously? Where was he a few days ago? Or ever? The soda samples looked and sounded so good, but I managed to keep walking. I'm glad I did because I happened to see bottles of seltzer water and stopped. Now if you don't know what seltzer water is, it is simply water with carbonation (aka the bubbles). While they do have flavors available, I opted for the plain grocery brand version for .99 cents. I went home and poured a glass and tried it. Wow, that was too strong. So I went to the fridge and pulled out lemon and lime juice and gave it a shot or two in my glass. Ahhhh. That hit the spot and immediately quenched my soda craving. Like flipping a switch, my brain canceled the nuke launches and depth com 5. I felt normal and I would reward myself after teaching my last CrossFit class each night by sitting down and quietly sipping the bubbly and cold drink. It was a perfect nightcap back then. But then one day, without noticing the transition, I stopped. The seltzer bottle in the fridge went flat and I never replaced it. My soda addiction was gone after nearly 20 years and I haven't touched a Dr. Pepper or soda since.

My headaches also disappeared over the next few days as my body and brain adjusted to having less sugar. You might be wondering how you can have sugar withdrawals if diet sodas do not have actual sugar. Artificial sweeteners have a more intense flavor than table sugar and increase a person's desire to eat even more sweet foods. Since I stopped buying a candy bar or donuts every time I bought a diet soda, I was actually coming off a small sugar high. It was a huge victory for me and the precursor to eventually beating my sugar addiction. I only wish I had been smart enough to realize that addictions never go away. They go quiet. They even pretend to be gone. The truth is they are waiting in the shadows. Waiting for a slip-up or laziness or perhaps a little of both. I fell for the trap about a year later when I came face to face with a monster.

I should mention at this same period in my life, I owned a CrossFit gym and taught most of the classes. Ironically, I would teach people how to get fit all through the day while I ate fast food and Subway sandwiches in between classes. I told myself I was too busy to stop and eat something better. At 5'8" and 180 pounds, I didn't look obese and my habits went unnoticed by the athletes I trained. Like a lot of Americans, I tried to make healthier choices overall and living with Amanda, a dietitian, was certainly a plus. Yet, no matter what I did or how many calories I counted, I would only drop a few pounds and then level off around 176. I wanted the weight loss and to literally eat my cake too. Despite Amanda beginning to caution me about my narrow view of "healthy", I continued to believe calories in versus calories out was the only way to effectively lose weight. It satisfied my desire to make my weight logical by reducing the complex issue of obesity into a numbers problem. I honestly thought that maybe given enough time, I could find the elusive perfect calorie count for me as if it was a magical number I hadn't discovered yet. Here is the truth: No such magical number exists. Calories are not created equal and 300 calories of a candy bar will have a much different impact on your body than 300 calories of leafy greens. I was trying to solve a quality equation with a specific quantity answer. It doesn't work that way. I understand that now, but at the time, I was struggling in quicksand. The more I wrestled with the problem, the faster I sunk.

In the fall of 2013, I had made the switch to non-carbonated energy drinks to help me stay awake during the day. I was recovering from shoulder surgery and only managing few restless hours of sleep each night. I can remember lying awake waiting for my alarm to go off at 4:30am so I could get up and not be in as much pain. By 3pm most days, I had to stop and take a nap because I had to be awake to teach the night classes. My drinks of choice were Monster Rehab and Rockstar Recovery which both have around 160mg of caffeine. For a reference point, a normal cup of coffee has roughly 95mg. The problem was, despite going from drinking one to two a day, the caffeine soon lost its kick and I was back to where I started. I could drink a full can and still fall asleep on the couch 5 minutes later. Ironically, I was also drinking a lot more added sugar than when I would only drink the Diet Dr. Peppers. In my attempt to get away from soda, I made my sugar addiction a lot worse. I drank the ultra-sugary energy drinks to help me stay away when in reality they were contributing to my inability to do so. It was a horrible cycle and all the while I was still giving myself kudos for counting my calories and not drinking soda.

Lucky for me, a new documentary came out in March of 2014 called "Fed Up" and the poster was adorned by a big "F U" on two M&M's. It was a documentary about the ill effects of added sugar. The narrator, Katie Couric, was researching the continuing climb of childhood obesity. By accident, they found the cause to be an absurd consumption of added sugars by the typical American family. Amanda and I played hooky one day and went to the local theater to see the film. We walked away talking about how the main issue wasn't that people simply didn't care if they were gaining weight, but like me, were horribly misinformed as to what was causing the repeated failures. I went home with renewed vigor and started researching sugar. I quickly found Robert Lustig's Youtube video "Sugar: The Bitter Truth" which had gone viral several months earlier and had over 6 million views. I became a fan of Dr. Lustig's work and listened to podcasts where he was the guest. Those early internet searches led to more articles and papers, and I began to see the link between added sugar and many of my eating habits. The light bulb turned on in my brain and all of a sudden I realized something profound: *I was a Sugar Addict.* 2 years later, the term still sounds awkward and a bit silly to me when I say it, but I find solace in reading the definition of addiction from the American Society of Addiction Medicine (asam.org):

Addiction is characterized by inability to consistently abstain, impairment in behavioral control, craving, diminished recognition of significant problems with one's behaviors and interpersonal relationships, and a dysfunctional emotional response. Like other chronic diseases, addiction often involves cycles of relapse and remission. Without treatment or engagement in recovery activities, addiction is progressive and can result in disability or premature death.

Let's see if that checks all the boxes for sugar. Inability to abstain? Yup, I could not stop eating food with sugar. Impairment in behavioral control? Cravings? A diminished recognition of significant problems? Yup, yup, and a big YUP. The last part though is the most striking. "Without treatment . . .addiction is progressive and can result in disability or premature death." That is in line with how Type 2 Diabetes starts and there are more and more studies coming out linking sugar to dementia, early-onset Alzheimer's, and non-alcoholic fatty liver disease, among many other diseases. My sugar addiction was killing me slowly and silently. I was on a direct path towards diabetes and that scared me. I knew something had to change, but I hadn't convinced myself it was all spiraling out of control.

On a family trip to Lexington, KY for Easter in late April, I came to terms with the extent of my problem. The candy, the breakfast pastries, and desserts were on each counter, table, and fridge shelf. I was like a madman and felt out of control. I remember making my dad a birthday cake that weekend and going back for a second and third piece. I even remember my brother looking over at me around 9pm when I was still eating cake and simply saying, "Damn Brian." I don't know how much sugar I consumed that weekend, but I went back home feeling disgusted and with a massive headache. It is one thing to feel bad and not understand why, but by this point, I knew exactly what was going on and I couldn't stop. I was depressed and the next few weeks were low points for me. It was a vicious cycle as I kept eating more cakes and candy trying to get rid of my cravings. Desserts and fast food were the only things that temporarily made me feel better. It was a cheap high and I knew it. Plus, I was at a point where no amount of cake or donuts were ever satisfying. I would get full, but that sugar craving would be back within hours and further down the rabbit hole I went.

Like most addicts, I finally hit rock bottom one Saturday morning when I brought home a donut for Sofia, who was 3 at this time. I wasn't mad I gave her a donut. It was that I gave a toddler a donut without her asking for one. What did I expect her to say? "No thanks Daddy. I don't want the donut you literally placed in front of me?" All at once, it seemed clear to me that my bad habits were already shaping how my daughter saw food and she was too young to know any different. The next day I sat down with Amanda and explained to her that if I kept going down this path, I was going to be sitting in doctor's office in the near future finding out that I was pre-diabetic or worse. At 36 years old, I had to accept that my current destructive behavior was now directly affecting my family. Sometimes you can reason that it is OK to destroy your own health, but I knew that morning that I was accepting Sofia as collateral damage. I said simply, "Starting tomorrow, I am giving up all added sugar." Amanda smiled at me and said, "OK, let's go food shopping tonight and I'll help you." To this day, I don't know if she honestly believed me or not. She never let on if she didn't. With her help and a renewed determination, May 19th, 2014 would be the first day of the rest of my life.

2 GROWING UP ON SUGAR

Looking back on that first grocery store visit, I can tell you I was experiencing a great deal of anxiety. I am a little embarrassed to admit this, but I walked through the aisles with a lump in my throat. I wasn't about to cry over my lost crumb cake, but the stress of the situation was intense. It is no wonder though since I was basically saying goodbye to a big and important part of my life. What did I turn to when I was sick or stressed or angry? Foods with lots of added sugar. What was an integral part of every holiday for the past 36 years? Added sugar. What was in most of the food I was eating even if I didn't consider them desserts or treats? Added sugar.

As a child of the eighties, my addiction or love of sugar was a huge part of my life. In fact, a year before I was born in 1978, the McGovern Report published data that villainized saturated fats. These findings are now widely discredited, but at the time, the report had a lot of muscle and launched a 30-year movement to lower fat intake. Nobody was talking about it then, but the best way to make food taste tolerable without fat is to add lots of sugar. So while we were all dutifully following the government's advice and eating less fat, our added sugar consumption soared. Around the same time, tougher sugar import taxes and the rise of corn subsidies made high fructose corn syrup (HFCS) the cheaper alternative to table sugar. It was now even easier to remove fat and add sugar substitutes. Food companies seized this opportunity to give the people exactly what they asked for; less fat. By 2010 when I was 32 years old, American adults were eating 30% (and children 20%) more calories from added sugar per day than when I was born in 1978.

I grew up on Long Island, NY. Our extended family on both sides lived somewhere between 20 minutes and 2 hours away. In fact, at one point, two of my uncles and my grandfather worked for a popular northern bakery called Entenmann's. The white boxes with blue cursive writing that they brought home were staples around our houses. I have fond memories of quiet mornings spent at my grandparent's summer home in Mattituck, NY. The boxes were scattered around the table on the screen porch. Breakfast always seemed to last for hours as the adults would often get up first and the cousins lagging behind. Like a lot of people, I fondly look back on this part of my childhood and the food that we ate together.

I was a normal American child of the 80's and 90's who loved sweets as much as the next kid. I wasn't obese though. I was fortunate to be active in karate for years and my mom did her best to put a healthy meal on the table each night. As the fat-free movement gained traction, my beloved blue and white boxes now had a new option with a yellow band around the corner. It proudly stated "Fat Free."

One article from 1994 said the company went from 12 fat-free options in 1989 to over 70 by 1994. Which looking back it is a wonder most of the fat-free food didn't taste much better. Think about it. They took out the fat, replaced it with lots of added sugar, and the best they could muster up was "palatable". Not to mention all the other chemicals they probably had to add to the food in order to make it stable.

My family dutifully chose the yellow bands over the plain boxes because it was the healthier choice. There was no reason to look beyond the front of the box. We were like a lot of other middle-class families in America. We ate the fat-free food, we replaced our butter with margarine, we dropped to 2% milk, and we ate a lot of Rice-A-Roni. OK, maybe that last one was only my family, but all I'm saying is we should have bought some stock in that San Francisco treat. After all, why would the government or the food industry intentionally deceive or lie about our health? Trust me, I'm not a conspiracy theorist by a long shot, but at that time we simply did not have the vast information machine known as the internet. If Dan Rather reported on it and the government backed it, that was good enough for my parents. By my graduation from high school in 1996, my sugar addiction had taken hold and was about to get a whole lot worse.

Let's fast forward a bit. After college, I found myself in Georgia working as a firefighter for Dekalb County. It was a great job and learning experience for the five years I stayed there. I spent most of my time at Station 23 in Clarkston, Ga which had roughly 12 firefighters on shift at any one time. As a rookie, I learned fast that you either responded "yes" or "no" when a senior firefighter asked at 7am whether you were in for dinner. God help you if you were stupid enough to ask what the ladder crew was planning on cooking. I don't know who started this tradition, but I do know those dinners and other big meals quickly caused me to gain weight like no other time in my life. I went from dropping 30 pounds to roughly 163 lbs before my wedding following Nutrisystem and eating their shelf-stable foods, to quickly topping 200 pounds within a year. Yes, I put on over 40 pounds in 1 YEAR. I would tell you exactly how much I topped out at, but the truth is I don't know. The last time I stepped on the scale back then it read 199 and I figured there was no use in continuing to look. So I didn't. If I went to the doctors, I looked away from the scale. Like a scared child, I figured if I didn't see it, it wasn't actually true.

Life got busy as Amanda and I both tackled our masters' degrees and nutrition took a back seat to the chaos. I know now that I gained a lot of weight during that period, but I didn't recognize it as a major issue at the time. I figured when I finished school and my life was less hectic, I would reign in the weight gain. Amanda was going to school to become a registered dietitian, but her course work still emphasized it was a calories in / calories out problem. She even had a shirt that said, "It is the calories, stupid" that she got from a national dietetics convention. With my weight gain picking up speed, I decided I couldn't wait to start making a change. I tried to follow along with Amanda's course work and only became more confused. I didn't know what to eat. I would try to make better choices, but even the healthy stuff didn't seem to make a difference. Nothing tasted sweet unless it was M&M's or cake and even those once beloved treats were starting to lose their power over my happiness. By the time Amanda and I finished our masters' programs, it was late 2008 and I was the heaviest I had ever been and depressed. To make matters worse, on August 8, 2008, my mom lost a hard fought battle with breast cancer. That night we sat as a family and watched the opening ceremony to the Beijing Olympics. In the quiet of that moment, I knew things were about to change in my life.

Within two months, Amanda accepted a job in Tampa and I said goodbye to Atlanta after nearly 30 years of calling it home. Then in 2009, I accepted a job as a contract firefighter in Iraq and spent the next 15 months there. It was on a base called Camp Falcon that I first learned about CrossFit and quickly fell in love with the simplicity of the training and how quick the workouts could bring me to my knees. It didn't take long for me to realize I was meant to bring CrossFit back to our small town in Central Florida and we opened U R CrossFit in early 2011. Two months earlier, we welcomed Sofia into our family and just like that we had a new baby and a new business. In the years to come, I would jokingly say I had two kids: Sofia and U R CrossFit. I share all of these experiences with you, the good and the bad, because they shaped who I was walking into the grocery store on May 18th, 2014 with Amanda. At the time, I had no idea if I would make it one day, let alone be writing a book about it two years later. All I knew back then was something had to change. It was now or never.

3 BEATING THE ADDICTION

I had my work cut out for me at that first grocery store visit. Especially since an estimated 75% of all foods in a grocery store have added sugar. If I was going to beat my life-long addiction, I felt it had to be drastic. With Amanda's help, we read a lot of packages, tried to stick with real foods that didn't have labels, and kept checking our phones to look up yet another name for added sugar, MSG's, and trans-fats. This ultimately allowed me to have enough food to eat for a few days. My grocery bag had steak, chicken, beef, lots of fruit, some vegetables, and potatoes. My initial goal wasn't even to eat balanced meals. I figured I would tackle that task down the road. I simply wanted to start eating foods without added sugar and get my life back on track. People often ask me if I started this plan to lose weight. Honestly, my weight was an afterthought because I felt like if I concentrated on this one big goal, perhaps my weight would drop. Lucky for me, quitting all added sugar does help with weight loss, and within a year, my body fat percentage had dropped from 22% to 14% without stepping on a scale once. Unlike my days on Nutrisystem where I lost 3 pounds per week, quitting added sugar had a much healthier pace and one day I realized my body looked completely different in the mirror. It didn't happen overnight, but my body was slowly showing all of the positive effects of getting rid of sugar.

So let me back up a second here and tell you how I decided to define added sugar. I decided I would no longer eat any real or fake sugars that were added to a food or showed up in an ingredient list. So real sugars like honey, maple syrup, and agave were out. Sugar substitutes like stevia and aspartame were also out. Fruit in its whole form was and still is totally fine. Fruit juice or any method where real fruit was crushed, squeezed, pulverized or otherwise to get the sweet juice was also considered added sugar. Why? Because fruit has natural fiber that buffers the rapid intake of natural sugar and often tells our brain when we are full and should stop eating. Fruit juices or concentrates do not. By default, these terms also meant I would be cutting out almost all processed foods and fast foods since most of them have added sugar in some form.

During this time, I decided not to count my calories and I still don't two years later. I was a huge fan of the app MyFitnessPal for a long time, but I realized that only counting calories was not going to tell the whole story. Plus, I figured that by eliminating all processed foods, all fast foods, all soda or sugary drinks, and of course, all food with added sugar listed in the ingredients list, the quality of my calories was going to be superior. This turned out to be one of the smarter things I did because it finally freed me of using inefficient tools like the scale and calories to define my success. What I did focus on was how I looked in the mirror. I took pictures and I compared. On days when I felt defeated or worn down, I would simply compare the earlier pictures with the recent ones and I had all of the ammo I needed to keep on fighting.

I also decided to get my blood work done at 3 months, 6 months, 12 months and 20 months after giving up added sugar. I compared these results to blood work I had done about a year earlier in 2013. These markers tell part of a bigger story that I believe would have lead me to being diagnosed with diabetes and other diseases.

	1yr prior	3 mths	6 mths	12 mths	20 mths
Total Cholesterol	245	202	184	181	180
LDL	168	138	115	117	110
HDL	55	47	54	54	57
Triglycerides	112	84	74	51	60
Total to HDL	4.5	4.3	3.4	3.4	3.5
Apo B	129		103		93
Lp(a)	18				19
Hs-CRP)	5.86		.7		.7

Insulin			1.5		
Hemoglobic A1c	5.9		5.7		5.4
Glucose	89	89	83	81	81
Blood Pressure	132/ 74				113/ 72
Resting Pulse	87				52
Weight	187	178	167	163	163
Waist in inches	36	34	33	32	30

To put these numbers into perspective, here are pictures of me from around those times.

2008 at my heaviest

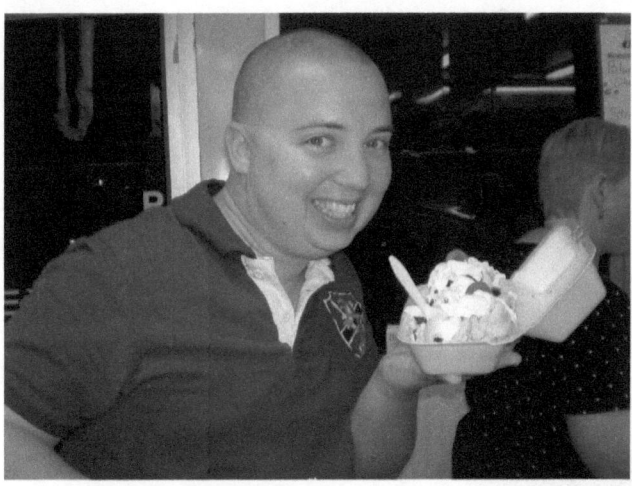

June 2013

(one year prior to giving up added sugar)

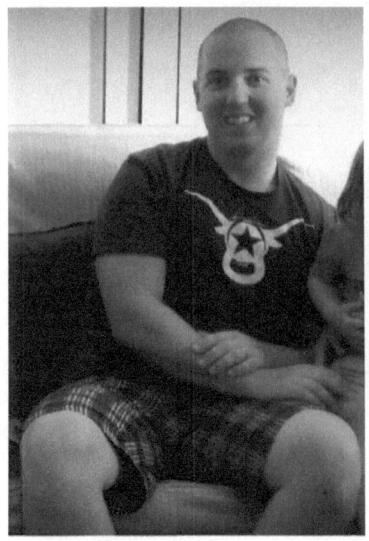

February 2015

(9 months after quitting)

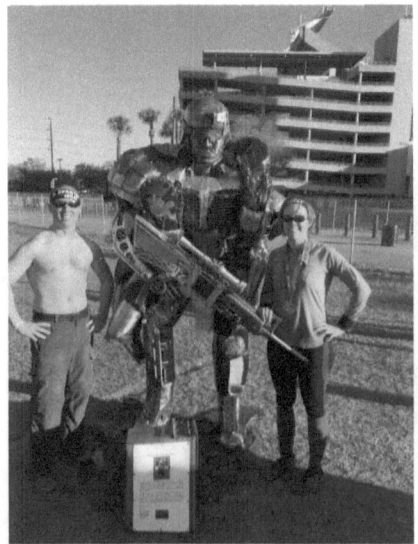

May 2015

(taken at the 1-year mark)

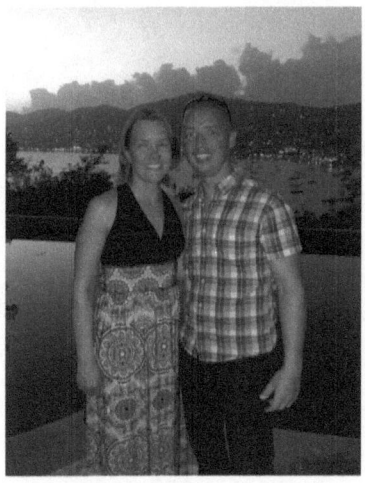

To see Amanda's and my fun take on a music video from this trip, go watch https://youtu.be/qbq06mTkfME.

November 2015

(18 months after)

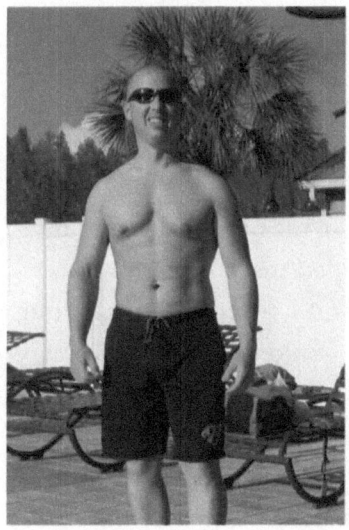

March 2016 (20 months)

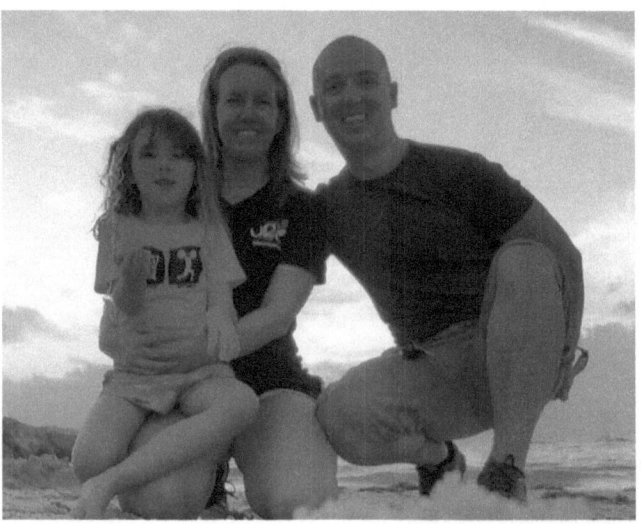

Finally, I want to mention working out. Despite owning a CrossFit gym and teaching in it several hours a day, I found it difficult to work out. Mainly because I refused to work out with my clients (that wasn't what they paid me for) and because the minute I was done with classes, I got out. The gym was my office and I don't know anybody who likes to hang around when they aren't working or getting paid. I mention this because I don't want to give the impression that I was working out a lot prior to giving up added sugar. Truthfully, my initial intention was to start working out three times a week once I began eating better, but that quickly unraveled. I found the stress of fitting in workouts while making changes to my diet that much harder. So I ultimately decided that nothing was as important as fighting my sugar addiction and I stopped working out. I told myself that I needed to prove that I could go 1 year without eating added sugar before I worried about adding working out to the mix. For some people, working out is a stress reliever but that was never the case for me. I needed to have less stressors in my life so that all of my attention and focus could be placed squarely on fighting the 800 pound gorilla in the room. With a few false starts under my belt, I finally got back into CrossFit for myself when we sold our gym after 5 years as owners. Today, I am finally enjoying the process of getting stronger and I can see the results in the mirror and how my clothes fit. Being active is an important part of being fit, but I am so glad I decided to concentrate on quitting added sugar because now I can say without a doubt that while working out is important, it is not even close to the importance of having a quality nutrition plan. I continue to take pictures and use the mirror as my primary guidance. The scale sits unused under our bathroom counter and MyFitnessPal had to go find a different pal to hang out with.

PART II

4 GOING SHOPPING AND THE FIRST TWO WEEKS

One of the most important ideas for me to convey with this book is that getting rid of added sugar in your life does not have to be overly complicated. With that in mind, the remainder of this book is about how I went through the actual process and the tools that you can use to do the same. Once I decided that I was going to quit, I needed to go shopping for food. I have discussed the emotional side of this trip, but not what I actually bought. While I have greatly expanded my variety of foods since those first trips to the store, below is an account of what I bought and ate early on as well as the price breakdown.

Food Record for Week One

5 Breakfasts:

Banana wrapped in a tortilla spread with peanut butter.

1 Tortilla Wrap from Whole Foods. The 365 brand has no added sugar

1 Organic Banana

1 tablespoon of fresh ground peanut butter.

8 Lunch and Dinners:

Either a burger or a steak and potato.

For the burgers, I used the best ground beef I could find at the store, then I would buy Ezekiel muffins to use as the bun. I topped my burgers with avocado and pepper jack cheese. I kept the steaks simple with basic spices and used butter and cinnamon on the sweet potatoes.

2 additional lunches or dinners:

Whole Foods Fresh Pizza.
I got lucky and found that our local Whole Foods made their pizza dough in house and it surprisingly did not have any added sugar in it or the sauce. It was basic and handy to have around.

Snacks:

Pre-chopped fruit and Nuts and Seeds

I ate a lot of fruit during my first two weeks. I didn't try to curb it either. I figured if I was craving something sweet, I would eat fruit until the craving went away. I made sure to only eat whole pieces of fruit so that my body had a chance to tell my brain it was full. When I wasn't eating it, I was constantly snacking on nuts and seeds. I didn't measure anything. I ate until I was satisfied. It wasn't long after that I realized how great being satisfied feels compared to hungry or overly-full.

Price break down for Week 1

Whole Foods 365 Traditional Tortillas 6pk	$2.19
5 Organic Bananas	$2.26
Publix Fresh Ground Peanut Butter	$3.20
4 Publix Mock Tender Grilling Steaks	$9.02
4 Organic Sweet Potatoes	$2.99
Publix Greenwise Ground Beef for burgers (1.2 lb)	$7.19
8 pack of Ezekiel Muffins for burger buns	$5.49
4 pack of individual Sabra Guacamole (Non-GMO Project)	$4.99
Cabot Pepper Jack Cheese bar (slice or shred it)	$3.89
Custom mix of nuts from Whole Foods	$10.00
Pure Leaf Unsweet Tea (64oz) I typically brew my own for less	$2.49
Whole Foods Fresh Small Cheese Pizza	$4.99
Large cut-up fruit bowls	$5.86
Total with Tax for 3 meals and snacks a day for 5 days	**$68.93**

So for about $4.50 a meal including snacks and drinks, you can eat mostly organic food with no added sugar for a week. If you want to do more. Great. If you want to spend less or more. Great. The point is you don't have to in order to give up added sugar. If you are inspired to do something now, take this with you to the store and buy exactly what I did. It takes a total of 10 minutes to buy it all and another 30 total minutes to cook the burgers, steaks, and potatoes. As a mentor of mine says, "Pursue simple. Get fancy later."

Food Record for Week 2

5 Breakfasts:

Banana wrapped in a tortilla spread with peanut butter.

1 Tortilla Wrap from Whole Foods. The 365 brand has no added sugar

1 Organic Banana

1 tablespoon of fresh ground peanut butter.

8 Lunch and Dinners:

Either spaghetti and meatballs or shredded chicken tacos

For the spaghetti and meatballs, I made sure I bought sauce without sugar added. I personally like the Monte Bene brand, but any sauce without sugar will do. Then I used simple spices like oregano, salt, garlic, and onion powder to mix in with the ground beef. 10 minutes on broil in the toaster oven and the meatballs are done. Total time for cooking is basically waiting for the water to boil for the pasta.

For the shredded chicken tacos, I started by boiling a few chicken breasts. Then I learned a trick where you put the cooked chicken in a mixer with the larger paddle attachment. Turn on the mixer and in about 3 minutes, the chicken is perfectly shredded. Otherwise, I used the same tortillas from the morning and use a bit of guacamole and any other veggies I have around and mix it with no sugar added salsa. There is no wrong way to make tacos though. Use the path of least resistance to get it done.

2 additional lunches or dinners:

Against the Grain Pizza.

These gluten free pizzas are made with tapioca starch and are found in the frozen section. They can be a life safer when you need a quick meal. I like the pesto and the cheese versions and I find a ¼ of the pizza is plenty for a lunch or light dinner.

Snacks: This depends on how you are feeling, but I stuck with mixed nuts and fruit. If that isn't enough variety, you can buy some tortilla chips or pretzels. Be sure to read the labels because they sneak added sugar in a lot of the products. Not to mention these options should be used sparingly as they are not the best source of carbohydrates.

Price break down for Week 2

Whole Foods 365 Traditional Tortillas 6pk x 2	$4.38
5 Organic Bananas	$2.26
Publix Fresh Ground Peanut Butter	$3.20
Publix Greenwise Chicken Breasts	$12.03
Monte Bene Sauce	$4.99
Publix Greenwise Ground Beef for meatballs	$8.39
Publix Pasta	$1.59
Against The Grain Frozen Pizza	$10.99
4 pack of individual Sabra Guacamole (Non-GMO Project)	$4.99
Pure Leaf Unsweet Tea (64oz) I typically brew my own for less	$2.49
Mini San Marzano Tomatillos	$3.99
5 Easy Peel Oranges for snacks	$2.88
Total with Tax for 3 meals and snacks a day for 5 days	**$62.18**

Like Week 1, I ate healthy food for about $4.50 a meal and didn't have to spend a ton of time in the kitchen. If you are still feeling uneasy about letting go of sugar, simply repeat this same two-week menu. That gives you a month of not having to worry about eating added sugar while your body and mind adjust. Trust me, making food prep a stress-free part of your life is essential to succeeding.

Preparing For The Worst

It is no secret that giving up added sugar comes with withdrawal symptoms. So I wanted to touch on how I felt during the first week or two. Months after quitting, Amanda admitted to me that she was preparing for the worst when I decided to cut added sugar. We were both aware of how much I was eating and she rightfully believed I might be curled up in the fetal position by day 3. Luckily, that was not the case and I did reasonably well the first week. While I did experience fatigue and headaches, I believe I helped myself by eating a lot of diced fruit. The nice thing about eating whole fruit was I could only eat so much before my brain told me to stop. True, I consumed a lot of natural sugar in the form of fructose that first week, but I also consumed the other nutrients and fiber that went with it. I remember sitting down at least twice a day with the bowl in front of me and just eating pieces of fruit until I felt full. Then I would put the bowl back in the fridge and do it again later. I honestly believe eating fruit helped offset any major headaches and I lost my desire to eat as much by the beginning of the second week. So fruit provided a temporary fix that probably saved me a lot of aches.

One area I did suffer a bit in was brain fog. I had a hard time during that first week remembering simple words and phrases. One time while teaching the 10am CrossFit class, I stood at the front of the gym explaining the workout and could not remember the word "jump." It wasn't there. No matter how long I tried to come up with it, I simply could not remember the world. I actually had to do it for one of my athletes who finally call out, "You want us to jump?" I said "YES. Thank you" and everyone laughed. The brain fog happened to me on several other occasions as well. I can't explain it other than to say that I didn't have the problem before I quit sugar and it didn't happen again after day 4 or 5.

Finally, I want to let you know that I didn't make a whole lot of plans during those first few weeks and I don't suggest you do either. I had nothing to do other than teach classes. I think I would have had a much harder time if other life events were happening along the way. So my advice is to go do the simple shopping first and prepare for the worst. Clear your schedule and be OK with relaxing a bit when you can (with your bowl of fruit).

5 SUGAR SYSTEMS

Within about two weeks of quitting, I realized I would need a few systems in place if I had any chance of succeeding and making my one-year goal. I knew the more organized I was, the better off I would do. Unlike cigarettes and alcohol that cannot be sold in certain places, sugary food has zero restrictions, and worse, it is actually geared towards kids which means an adult has no chance of avoiding it. There was no food store, gas station, or frankly any other type of store that wouldn't at the very least have a gumball machine or a display with candy bars on it. Sugar is low cost, high yield, and makes for a great impulse buy at checkout. So unless I was planning to only sit inside my house and not work or run errands for my family, I was going to have to be around the one thing I was trying to avoid. I needed a written plan that I could refer back to. I called these plans the Sugar Systems.

The No-Go Zones

My first system was to plot spots in town that were deemed "no-go" and I told myself to avoid them. It was a system and it was organized and it saved me from getting myself into a bad situation where I might be tempted to make poor choices. For example, I had a habit of getting a Monster Rehab drink and a Dunkin Donut (or three) from the local Hess station when I needed gas. So in order to not put myself in that situation, I would only get gas after I had eaten a meal and was less likely to want to binge on sugar. I also made sure that I always paid at the pump and never walked into the convenience store. The only thing in there that was convenient was rapid ingestion of sugar, so it became a "no-go" zone. Another example of a no-go was all fast food restaurants even if I thought they had food available that didn't have added sugar. For instance, you can get unsweetened iced tea from Starbucks and McDonalds, but I told myself there were probably other ingredients in the drink that I didn't want or need such as caramel coloring. Beyond the obvious, I also considered some bars off limits because they served beer that might contain added sugars. Fortunately, this was an easy choice because we had a craft beer brewery down the street and I could actually watch the beer being made.

Having no-go zones in place will save you when you are stuck out somewhere, get hungry, and you have nothing around you to eat. Guess how fast you will start making excuses why it is OK to eat at McDonald's this one time? You start telling yourself you didn't mean to stay out past lunch and the world happened and you were a victim. I've been there. Those thoughts drove me crazy sometimes and I would get angry how it was unfair that I had this problem and others didn't. Instead, I encourage you to map out your own "no-go" locations before trying to give up added sugar. A little prep work up front does go a long way towards success and it is super easy to keep a Zip-lock bag of nuts and seeds in your car for those unplanned situations. If nothing else, plotting out these zones will open your eyes to the amount of unknown added sugar in your community.

My 5-Step Shopping System

While getting around town and avoiding added sugar was difficult, nothing seemed as daunting as going back to the scene of the crime. A grocery store for a sugar addict is like a cigar bar for a smoker. The smells and fumes are all around and my brain knew it. So having a system in place for shopping was a necessity. I should mention that when I gave up added sugar, I went cold turkey and literally switched over night. Even with Amanda for support, it was still stressful. Since I don't advocate this sudden stop, I developed a system for slowly eliminating added sugars over time. Regardless of the route you chose, following these steps will help get you in and out of the store quickly and with little to no stress.

My advice is to take your time, go in with a full stomach, read lots of labels, and don't worry about the lack of diversity in your food. So what if you are going to eat a piece of steak for the first 3 nights and have plain yogurt with strawberries for breakfast for the entire first week? Your initial goal is to avoid added sugar. My advice is to get the first two weeks planned out like I did and only concentrate on the basics. Once you have a month under your belt, I recommend using this 5 step process to navigate the store efficiently. Remember, this is a lifestyle change, not a diet. There is no one quick fix solution. This process will allow you to make slow, but constant improvements that won't stress you out.

Step 1: Establish your route

Like I mentioned earlier, 75% of the food in a typical grocery store have added sugar. That might seem overwhelming, but you can make it work for you. Think of it this way: You only have to look at 15% now. You need to establish a route and follow it. I pick up food in the same order on each trip. I don't wander. Wandering leads to the bakery. Always! At my local grocery store, the bakery is off in the front right corner as I walk in and the produce section is behind it in the back right corner. So when I walk in, I head straight for produce. In fact, I can tell you the first five things I pick up on a typical trip from habit and doing it so many times: Guacamole, bananas, grape tomatoes, unsweetened apple sauce, and grapes. Not only is this incredibly efficient, it reduces the stress of being overwhelmed by the thousands of food items lining the shelves and calling your name. From produce, I head along the back wall and pick up any meats or dairy I need. When get to an aisle I need, I duck in quickly and grab only what I am there for and get back on track. On the other side of the store I grab frozen fruits and vegetables from the freezer section, some mixed nuts, beer on occasion, and I'm out the door. Of course your local store might be completely different, but your goal should be the same. Establish a route and stick to it.

Step 2: Only buy USDA Organic and Non-GMO Project

Here is an easy way to narrow down your no added sugar choices. Only buy items that are labeled USDA Organic or Non-GMO Project. Why? Both labels have been independently verified by Consumer Reports as being the most trustworthy. Don't kid yourself. Plenty of these products still contain added sugars. The idea here is to further limit the amount of foods you actually need to look at. If you have a wall of pasta sauce in front of you and you are starting to sweat, only focus on the food with one or both of these labels on it. In my store, the price tags in front are now green, so it is even easier to quickly identify the USDA Organic or Non-GMO Project foods. Oh and don't worry about the added cost. I have found I always come out ahead because I am no longer buying stuff I don't need. No waste equals reduced costs and will easily make up for the added cost of going organic or GMO free.

Step 3: If the ingredient list takes more than 10 seconds to read, put it back.

Once you find a new food organic or non-GMO food, you need to find the ingredient list and read through it looking for added sugars. Except, if you are like me, you don't have 20 minutes to dissect the entire nutrition label and ingredients list. So I came up with a quick rule. If there are more words there than I can read in about 10 seconds, I put it back. Nothing you need to eat has that many ingredients. In fact, some of my favorite foods have 7 or less ingredients. My point is there are other healthier fish in the sea. Throw this one back. You will notice that many of the organic food labels seem longer because they often have to use the word "organic" before each ingredient, but you should still be able to quickly run through the list and reasonably identify all ingredients.

Step 4: Avoid J.O.S.S.

You are now looking at a smaller ingredient list and you want to know if it has added sugar. Well, there are now well over 60 different names for added sugar. Got time to memorize them all? Me neither. Instead, simply remember the acronym J.O.S.S which stands for Juice, -Ose, Sugar, and Syrup. If the food you are looking at has juice, words ending in -ose (like sucrose), sugar, or syrup in the name, it has added sugar. Avoid these ingredients and find another choice.

Step 5: Swap 1 item per grocery trip

At this point, you should have 1 solid choice in your hand that is remarkably better than whatever you used to buy. For example, you typically buy Ragu Pasta Sauce with lots of added sugar and sodium, and now you have Organico Bello Marinara with half the sodium, no added sugar, and only 8 ingredients. Great! Stop there. Pat yourself on the back and don't try to find more food swaps unless you have time to kill. You can obviously do it like I did and try to cut out all added sugar in one shopping trip, but I will tell you it is an unpleasant experience and I wouldn't do it again. Learn from my mistakes.

The quick math shows that in only 2 months, you would have found 16 new products you didn't know existed before. Think about that. We are creatures of habit and most of us already have a limited scope when it comes to the food we eat. I know some people who literally eat the same foods on the same day each week much like Sheldon Cooper from the Big Bang Theory. Taco night is always taco night. I like a bit more variety and I have found that if I can come up with two separate two-week meal plans, I am rarely getting bored with the same food. I must stress though that this takes time. If you try to do it right out of the gate, you will fail. It is overwhelming enough to quit added sugar without having to plan for that many meals. Take my advice and follow the 5 steps above. At first you will be eating a lot of the same things, but that quickly changes and before you know it, you are living a different nutrition lifestyle. You are not on a diet. Diets mean temporary and that is not your goal. Small changes you make today are potential life-savers tomorrow. Don't underestimate the power of what you are accomplishing and give yourself a lot of credit for taking these first steps.

My System for Eating Out

In the month or two right after I started changing my lifestyle, I was focused on playing by my own rules and staying on top of the food I ate. It is actually easier at the beginning because, presumably, you have not found that many foods that fit into your new regimen. So while the limits of variety may be boring, there is a lot to say for boring being safe too. One of the slight mistakes I made early was being a little too rigid when it came to going out and eating. As you would imagine, finding any food without added sugar can be hard to come by in a typical American restaurant. At first, I would eat a steak and baked potato because it was an easy choice. If the restaurant didn't have steak and potatoes, we went somewhere else. Since I don't care for salads, I started to wonder if I could eat other menu items like a burger. The problem is most bread has added sugar in it. While I was able to eventually find a restaurant that did make their own bread with no sugar, I would typically resort to a bun-less burger wrapped in lettuce. Here is the problem with that idea. While it has all of the ingredients of a good burger, wrapping a slab of beef in lettuce does not make a burger. It makes a warm salad sandwich. My point is, it was horrible. OK, maybe that is too harsh. It was horrible. Yeah, see I can't even get myself to write something better.

What I should have done was had a better system to deal with eating out in the first place. After trying it once, I should have realized it wasn't tasty to me or met my standards for happiness, and never ordered it after that. "Almost tastes like" is not a long term solution to any new lifestyle. It frankly makes you mad that you can't have something you want. Another good example of this was when Amanda made "ice cream" by whipping frozen bananas. Now, I like bananas. I used to eat one with peanut butter most morning. However, frozen whipped bananas are 1. not ice cream, and 2. not remotely good. The moral here is don't eat substitutions that don't satisfy your craving for the original food. Life is too short to be eating stuff you don't like when there are literally hundreds of foods or meals that you do like and are perfectly healthy. You might have to look a little harder to find them if you are a picky eater like me. Try new foods once or twice, but be completely OK with never trying it after that. Instead, take those opportunities to try something new like sweetbread. If you ever meet me, ask me about the time I had this meal that is neither sweet, nor bread. Sometimes being adventurous pays off and sometimes it is sweetbread. You have to take the good with the bad.

Not Getting Too Comfortable

Another mistake I made along the way was actually finding too many foods that didn't have added sugar in them. Let's take Lay's Original Potato Chips for example. They have about five ingredients in them and none of them are sugar. I found myself eating an increasing amount of small bags of Lays. Why? Perhaps because I could. I'm not sure. I just know I got lazy, I found a loophole, and I sort of ran with it. The problem is loopholes don't equal healthy options. What I did to correct this was I simply identified the issue, went and found other healthier snacks, and made the switch. Simple and effective. Luckily, I have no addiction to chips, so the correction was quick and harmless. Be careful that you don't take advantage of the loopholes. You need a system in place to identify these "grey-area" foods and decide at the beginning how you will deal with them. Because if you wait until you are hungry and are staring at the Lay's bag, you have little chance of making a rational decision. Don't get me wrong, one bag of chips on occasion is totally fine. However, it should not replace eating better options like mixed nuts. The only way this works though is if you define it and make the rules stick. I found writing them down and posting them on the fridge made the systems and rules feel more legit and I rarely had a problem sticking to them. Order is, after all, the opposite of chaos. And sugar loves chaos.

Here is the deal. You are going to mess up regardless of the systems you create. It is inevitable. And messing up doesn't have to mean falling off the wagon completely and the police finding your slumped against the wall at DQ with a blizzard in your hand and a frozen cookie dough ball rolling down your shirt. More than likely, it will be missteps that you maybe never saw coming like me and the potato chips. Regardless, remember you are the captain of your ship and this is not a diet. Let me repeat that. THIS IS NOT A DIET. Remember, you are making a lifestyle change and that means nothing is temporary except for the mistakes. Pick yourself back up, and go at it with even more determination. Develop your own systems and live by them. Allow them to make your life easier and efficient. A life without added sugar is worth the trials and tribulations early on because it gets easier over time. At the two-year mark, I barely have to think about what I will be eating today or for the rest of the week. I have so many options at my disposal that avoiding added sugar is actually pretty easy. Having systems in place is what will get you from day 1 to this point.

6 SNACKS

Ahh, the snack chapter. This one is my favorite, and let's be honest, a snack will save you more times than not when you are in one of those tricky situations. When I was a CrossFit gym owner, I didn't have a lot of time or space to make big meals in between classes. So I had to figure out a way to still get quality nutrition without having to resort to the typical sugar filled energy bars or snacks that were labeled as healthy but had 30 ingredients and 5 different types of added sugars.

My go to snack at the gym was always the same. Early on, I made a trip to Whole Foods and found that lovely wall of mixed nuts. At first, it seemed like a gold mine. Then you start reading labels and realize that half of it is adult candy dispensers and the other half have dried cranberries mixed in. Cranberries: The fruit nobody likes by themselves because they are super tart. You know how you fix tart? Lots of added sugar. So while the ingredient list might say cranberries, what they actually mean is cranberries + sugar to make them palatable. By the time I was done reading top to bottom and left to right along the great wall of nuts and candy, I found one winner. It was called "Strider's Snack" and it had raisins, almonds, cashews, hazelnuts, and walnuts. A few small handfuls during the day was enough to keep my hunger at bay and it never affected me while I was teaching. The only downside would be how much they get stuck in your teeth. The positive is you will drink a lot more water. So it is a win-win.

Now, raisins by design can be considered concentrated sources of sugar. They are dried grapes and grapes have higher levels of fructose in them. However, raisins in my mind are still whole fruits and I don't exclude them from the foods I eat. That being said, I am aware of how raisins can be abused so I only typically eat them if they are a part of mixed nuts or perhaps used as part of a topping. My suggestion with them or other fruits like dates is to use them sparingly and do some tests to see how your brain reacts. If you can eat a few raisins and you don't notice an increased desire to eat more sweet stuff, I would say you are probably ok. On the other hand, if you are like me, eating too many dates definitely makes my brain fire off and I imagine I would have a pretty significant dopamine response. So although they are fruit, you have to be careful. While I'm on the subject of dates, I definitely consider anything with mashed dates to be added sugar. Lara Bars and RxBars use crushed dates as a sweetener. They are cleverly marketed adult candy bars. Don't fall for the trap.

Owning a gym has its perks when it comes to finding out about new supplements and workout nutrition. We would get a box randomly in the mail with new bars or energy drinks in the hopes that we would give them to our members and maybe start selling them. The problem was most of it was junk. The supplements had "proprietary blends" and were typically loaded with one or several types of added sugars. So they were not a viable snack in terms of protein shakes or your typical gym shakes. Usually those follow up calls ended with me saying my wife was a dietitian and would be happy to discuss their ingredients. Click. Yeah, having standards is tough and it definitely cost us some income as gym owners, but the moral victory of not selling our members less than nutritious food always seemed to win out.

Not all were losers though. Amanda and I did find two different bars that we liked and still eat to this day. The first is called EPIC Bar. Here is how they describe them on their website, EpicBar.com. "EPIC bar is a 100% grass fed animal based protein bar designed as nature intended. Paleo friendly, gluten free, and low in sugar, we believe that EPIC foods should inspire EPIC health." The taste of an EPIC bar is like a softer beef jerky and we found our members at the gym were usually split on the taste. Those that liked them, loved them. Those that didn't, never tried a different flavor. I like them and they are excellent sources of animal protein.

The other bar we came to love is CORE. On their website, corefoods.com, they describe their snacks as "A delicious pack of hearty oatmeal ready to eat. Made with simple, powerful ingredients (no syrup, salt, flour, or oil). Free of preservatives and other additives, our food is perishable." The bars (meals) come in three flavors and two varieties: With and without organic whey protein. Both are great choices and I am a fan because they don't simply smash dates into their bars like I mentioned earlier. The company is also easy to like because they are a non-profit dedicated to feeding their community healthier options. I should mention here that I have no financial ties to either company and won't make a dime should you chose to buy them. Good snacks and portable food are hard to find when you are avoiding added sugar, so when I find the diamonds in the rough, I tell the world. Enjoy!

The mixed nuts, the Epic bars, and the Core Meals still do make up a good portion of the snacks I carry around with me. Other easy snacks are cut up fruit and healthier chips to dip in guacamole. Frankly, anything dipped in guacamole is fine by me. I eat it like it is going out of style. Be careful and read the ingredients first. You never know where added sugar might be lurking. Also, you might notice that most of my snacks are higher in good fats. Trust me when I say I eat a lot of fat. Guess what? Good sources of fat are good for you. My extensive blood work reflects that fact. Let's all have a moment of silence for the death of the low-fat craze. Good riddance.

7 THE POWER OF "NO"

Up to this point, I have told you how I became a sugar addict and how I started to create a lifestyle without added sugar. However, I have not told you the most powerful weapon I have. That is the power to say "no". Let me explain. Prior to quitting, I tried many different diets with varying levels of success. One of the more popular ideas was to eat healthy 80% of the time and not so healthy the other 20%. The idea being that if you are good for most of your life, the other small part will not matter. So I would eat healthy and then get to have a "cheat day" on Sunday. First of all, if you are changing your lifestyle, there are no cheat days. Second, I would fall off the wagon so hard on Sunday, that I would feel miserable on

Monday and have some sugar to make it better. I then would have a headache on Tuesday and have some sugar to make it better. If I was lucky, I would get back on track by Wednesday. So my cheat day typically lasted 3 days, and maybe if I wasn't too stressed out, I was eating clean for the other 4. I am amazed when I look back that I convinced myself I was doing good. Despite my best intentions, I found that as a sugar addict, it was a black and white world. So I simply decided to say "no." So what does saying "no" actually mean? Let's review my plan:

- I said no to all real or fake sugars that showed up in the ingredient list of any food. If it did not have an ingredient list, it was most likely a whole food like an apple, steak, or a carrot. Any sugar found in whole foods is there naturally and is not excluded.
- I said no to all fruit juices, fruit concentrates, or any other form of fruit that has been altered from its original form to make the sugar concentration greater. An example of this would be crushed dates that form a paste and are the main sugar source for some popular energy bars.
- I said no to any food with an ingredient list that took me longer than 10 seconds to read and I always bought a food that was USDA Organic or Non-GMO Project Verified whenever available.

Here is the important part: I said no to all of these things ALL of the time. I still do. I have never had a cheat day, a cheat meal, or even a single M&M since I began this journey. At the time of this book's writing, I have now gone almost two years and said no at each instance. And I know what some of you are thinking right now. "Wow, that sounds awful." I felt pretty bad for me too at the beginning. And perhaps you will never have to be as strict as me. I certainly know people who can take or leave sugar much like I can take or leave alcohol. If there were 5 years between my last beer and my next beer, I'd be fine with it. Unfortunately, my brain does not work like that with sugar. When I have even a small portion, something in my brain lights up like the Christmas tree in Rockefeller Center and I am off to the races. Will one single M&M cause this chain reaction? No. Probably not. Is it worth finding out? Definitely not. So I chose to do what has become the easiest and best part of this experience. I simply say "no".

What I believed would be the hardest part became my secret weapon. You know how you successfully go to Thanksgiving dinner and not eat any added sugar? You say no to the dressings and the pies and the sweet rolls. You know how you go out to eat and avoid foods with added sugar? You say no to choices that obviously have added sugar in them or you ask the waiter for clarification on the rest. Or when all else fails, have a steak and a baked potato. It is never "just this once". That means there is a choice to be made and choices create stress.

"No" is easy.

"No" is stress free.

"No" is the best part of this whole journey.

It is the surprise I found when I thought there were none. When you decide to say "no", you take the power away from the food, your friends and family, and the situation. As you will see in the next chapter, it also makes overcoming objections much easier.

8 FEELING GOOD ABOUT YOUR DECISION

When I first started eating better and avoiding sugar, I was concerned about social gatherings like birthdays, holidays, dinners at a friend's house and so on. My fear was that my family and friends would not take me seriously or perhaps they would simply not understand my addiction since they didn't have issues with sugar. After all, a sugar addict is not exactly a well-recognized term. To my knowledge, there are no SA meetings for sugarholics anonymous or well established support networks. So it was reasonable to assume I would get some push back simply from ignorance. While most of my family and friends were actually happy for me and wanted to know more about what I was doing, there are always a few who don't quite understand. For those that were intrigued or were interested in understanding why, I would give them the following answers. My hope is that they may help you one day as well.

Giving up added sugar is a lifestyle choice, not a diet.

"Diet" is one of those words that has been hijacked by for-profit organizations who are looking to make a fast buck on quick weight loss. Whereas it used to simply mean "The kind of food a person habitually eats" it is now more synonymous with the second definition which states, "A special course of food to which one restricts oneself, either to lose weight or for medical reasons." It is unfortunate, but a diet no longer represents my life. I live a sugar-free lifestyle. Unlike a diet, I have no end-game or point where I feel I will have succeeded. I don't care about losing any more weight and now my focus is simply on moving closer and closer to overall fitness and away from sickness. Yes, it is a lifestyle that I am happy to live and I do not believe I will change course anytime soon.

All carbohydrates break down into sugar, but not all carbohydrates are equal

While all carbohydrates do eventually break down into a simple sugar called glucose, there is a big difference between the quality of those carbohydrates, the rate of absorption, and the insulin response to them. So no, eating added sugar is not the same thing as eating any carbohydrate such as a sweet potato. With that said, I have found I feel even better when I do limit the amount of grains in my life. It is a choice backed by my own study of 1.

Added sugars speed up disease and rob you of nutrients

Several studies have labeled added sugars as non-nutrients which means you have a better chance of living on just water. In fact, there is a story in the book *Sugar Blues* by William Dufty (a great book written in 1975 about the history of sugar) where he talks about pirates being ship-wrecked on an island. He says given two groups of pirates, one group with water, and another group with water and sacks full of sugar, the pirates with only the water would likely live longer despite having no food. Why? Scurvy. If you are not familiar with the deadly disease from hundreds of years ago, it is caused by a deficiency of Vitamin C. It also turns out that Vitamin C and glucose (simple sugars) have common chemical structures and they compete for absorption by the cells. The higher the sugar consumption, the less Vitamin C can be utilized. So while both groups of pirates would undoubtedly suffer from lack of Vitamin C, the pirates consuming sugar would get there a lot faster. Not to mention refined sugar is void of vitamins and minerals which means it needs to draw upon the body's stores in order to be metabolized. So while some may look at added sugar as empty calories, I actually think the problem is much worse. Added sugar is robbing people daily of nutrients. I am no longer surprised when I see yet another report correlating the rise in disease and our increased consumption of sugar over the past 30 years.

I actually gave up a lot more than added sugar

Giving up added sugar certainly is the easiest thing to say, but this book could easily have been titled, "I am a Sugar Addict, a Processed Food Junkie, A Chemical Additive Connoisseur, and Lover of All Foods Not Found in Nature." Because added sugar is found in so many foods we eat, avoiding it means effectively avoiding a lot of other damaging ingredients. I may never know what ultimately brought my blood work to healthy levels aside from sugar. I'm OK with that. For me it doesn't matter if I could have achieved the same results forging a different path. There is simply no valid argument for attempting to do so when added sugar provides no benefits.

Giving up added sugar helped me to simplify my food choices for the better.

One of the benefits of reducing or eliminating added sugar is it takes a lot of other ingredients with it. For example, let's compare two different frozen pizzas that I used to buy. One that I used to eat prior to giving up added sugar, and one after the fact. The first is Kashi's Thin Crust Margarita Pizza. I used to eat it because Kashi is associated with being healthy and I figured it was better than Papa John's. Based on the ingredient label, there are a few different forms of added sugar. The crust has oat syrup solids and barley malt extract. The oat syrup solids are made by treating oats with acid and the barley malt extract is made by breaking down the barley and removing the fiber. The result for both is an added sugar used by Kashi to make the crust taste slightly more sweet. The sauce has cane juice solids which is another form of added sugar meant to look like a healthy option, but in reality is not that much different than table sugar. It also has maltodextrin which is typically found in candy and in Europe goes by the name, Glucose Syrup.

Now let's look at "Against The Grain's Pesto Pizza". I found this pizza at Whole Foods on one of my many shopping expeditions, but because it is gluten free, it has gained popularity and can now be found in my local grocery store. At least that is one positive from the gluten-free diet craze. Looking at the ingredient list, there are no added sugars to be found. The crust is made of tapioca starch, milk, canola oil, cheddar cheese, mozzarella cheese, and parmesan cheese. The topping is more cheese, water, canola oil, sunflower seeds, basil, and fresh garlic. I'm not a huge fan of canola oil and would prefer olive oil, but otherwise this pizza falls right in line with my no added sugar guidelines. There is, by the way, 1g of sugar in a serving of this pizza, but it is not added sugar. It comes from lactose in the milk used to make the cheeses.

By switching out the Kashi for the ATG pizza, I eliminated over 20 ingredients. They include natural flavors (no better than artificial flavors) and xanthan gum. I also got rid of the 4 types of added sugar that Kashi sprinkled through the ingredient list. Now I'm not claiming that those 20 ingredients were necessarily bad for me, but what positive effect could they have? In the years since quitting, I have found that foods with little or no ingredients taste the best. I will take a 5 ingredient drop biscuit any day over a Pillsbury Grand Biscuit with 30 or more ingredients. I am more satisfied and my body digests it better. That is a win-win for me.

9 GOOD FOOD WITH BENEFITS

My initial goal when I started was to simply stop putting added sugar in my system. It was basic and I purposely did not add a bunch of bells or whistles to my plan. I honestly did not have a desired weight I wanted to reach or a specific number for my cholesterol. I wanted to stop the cycle of unhealthy eating. Which is why all of the benefits I am about to tell you were all such a nice surprise.

- My sinus headaches disappeared: Prior to giving up added sugar, I would get seasonal allergies here in Florida that seemed to be getting worse with age. Of course, I carelessly brushed this off to getting older and convinced myself adult-onset allergies was a real thing. Within 1 week of giving up added sugar, my headaches disappeared. No more excruciating pain over my eye. No more Sudafed. No more anything. They all disappeared. I wasn't allergic to pollen or other seasonal plants. I was allergic to unhealthy food. Prior to giving up added sugar, if I didn't take a Sudafed, I would often be laying on the couch around 3pm with a washcloth over my eyes because the bright light always made the headaches worse. By 7pm the headaches would go away as if they were punching a timecard on the day shift. This would go on for weeks at a time and I was miserable. Now I cannot prove that sugar alone was my true intolerance because I had also given up processed foods, fast foods, and a lot of chemicals by default. It doesn't matter though. Getting rid of added sugar saved me from a lot of pain and headaches.

- My bathroom routine also got a lot easier: Now, I'm trying to be PC here, but I think we all know that poor food choices lead to more time in the bathroom. I didn't know I had an issue here until I didn't. Let's just say my days of running to a bathroom because my body was rejecting something I ate came to a quick and pleasant halt.

- My overeating habit stopped. I honestly had no idea how much I tended to overeat and get an unpleasant full feeling. You know what I mean. Like when you eat too much pasta and sauce, load up on garlic bread, and still tell yourself you want dessert because God knows you might never see a piece of cake for the rest of your life. The kind of full that instantly makes you want to lay down and take a nap. I'm happy to report those fun meals are a thing of the past. It turns out when you eat real food and dessert is no longer an option, you stop right about the time your brain tells you to. I can count on one hand how many times I have overeaten in the past year and a half. Each time I think to myself, "I can't believe this awful feeling used to be part of my life." Here is the truly depressing part. It was all self-inflicted pain. I had been doing it so long I think I actually believed it was normal to eat like that, feel stuffed, have a run to the bathroom, and then want to pass out for 20 minutes on the couch.

- My sleep pattern and energy got better: Getting rid of added sugar for me is like somebody deciding to charge my batteries all the way up to 100%. It is no coincidence that our business started to take off right around the time I stopped added sugar. Many of my athletes mentioned how I seemed much happier, more attentive, and had a renewed energy while teaching classes. It is no stretch to say cutting added sugar for me actually lead to greater financial success. If you had asked me before my lifestyle change, I would have told you I had plenty of energy and felt fine. The problem is you don't know what fine or good or even great is until the fog clears. When I mentor people, the hardest part is getting them to believe that what they are currently experiencing isn't normal and that the alternative is so much better. I live for the days when I get a call or email from one of my athletes saying they cannot believe how much better they feel on a no added sugar lifestyle.

- My taste buds can taste naturally sweet foods. This actually happened within about two weeks of giving up the added sugar. Once I gave my tongue a break, it rewarded me with a different, and enhanced, taste of sweetness. It is well documented that when you consume a lot of added sugar or even artificial sweeteners, you get desensitized to natural sweetness from fruit and other foods. For me, there was nothing sweet about grapes or strawberries for most of my life. When Amanda would mention to me that a farm picked strawberry was sweet, I would typically say that M&M's were sweet, but strawberries were sort of plain tasting and boring. That all changed pretty quickly and now I love strawberries and sometimes find them too sweet. Go figure.

- My teeth aren't horrible. This leads me to another great discovery which is I actually don't have horrible teeth lovingly passed down to me from my mom and dad. True, some dental history is genetic, but I now know most, if not 99%, of the problems I was having were of my own doing. Since quitting added sugar, I have had zero issues at the dentist. Talk about putting money back in your pocket.

- My weight and overall body image changed drastically: I had no expectations going in, so the fact that my entire body looks different now is a great surprise. I went from a starting weight of 178 and almost two years later I am holding at approximately 163 pounds and 12% body fat. Now when I put on weight, I know it is from being in the gym and working out. The vain side of me doesn't mind being able to see the outline of my abs in the mirror either. Because that is a sign that I am doing things the right way.

- My daughter is healthier. One of my mistakes was believing that my daughter (3 at the time) would have a hard time adjusting to not going to fast food restaurants like McDonald's and Chic-fil-A. Not only did Sofia adapt quicker than I did to not eating as much added sugar, but she quickly developed a distaste for sweeter foods. Today, she is 5 and actually makes her own videos about the dangers of added sugar for other kids. She has also completed an entire Whole30 challenge with Amanda and I which is an elimination plan where you don't eat grains, dairy, added sugar, legumes, or drink alcohol for 30 days. When her teachers asked her what she was doing, she said "I am trying to see what foods I am sensitive to." I am a proud dad.

Perhaps you are the main cooker in your house and you worry about the push back from family if you cut out added sugar. There are two ways to look at this. You can do what I did and eventually find a meal delivery service like Trifecta Nutrition that delivers healthy, organic, no added sugar, meals to your door weekly. It might cost more, but it will save you a lot of time cooking and cleaning up. This in turn results in more time with family and less in the kitchen. The other option of course is to bring your family along for the ride. Sure there is bound to be some uproar about the change, but you will never have to worry if taking added sugar away from the family table and kitchen was a healthier option.

If you are reading this book and seriously contemplating giving up added sugar, the reality is you have no idea all the ways it will make your life better. It isn't all about vanity, but I have never shied away from that being an important part of it all. How you look has a tremendous impact on how you feel, so I never discredit or make fun of anybody who simply wants to "look better." After all, a great way to start the day is to wake up, walk to the bathroom, look at yourself in the mirror naked and actually be happy with what you see. It is like somebody giving you an award daily for doing the right thing. Plus, it doesn't hurt for relationships either. My wife isn't exactly upset I don't eat donuts anymore.

10 YOUR ACTION PLAN

You have heard my story, but what about yours? After reading this book, do you consider yourself a sugar addict like me? Perhaps you recognize the immense health benefits of giving it up but don't think you are actually addicted. Either way, if this book has inspired you to begin to avoid added sugar, than I want to provide you with the best action plan I can for success.

Step 1: You Have to be Ready to Change

This book is all about how I finally committed to change and made it stick. What it doesn't go into a lot of detail about are all the times I tried Paleo, Zone, diets based on calorie restriction, cheat days, 80/20 rules, or other means of losing weight and failed. Not necessarily because the nutrition plans were bad either. I failed because I was never emotionally ready to begin with. I went in with the mindset of losing weight and success defined as reaching some mythical target weight that was going to make life wonderful.

Here is a good analogy: Sometime around 2003 I was single and sitting around a table with my cousins. I'm not sure how the conversation came up, but at some point I said, "I think I will be engaged within two years." Well the roar of laughter from my all-girl first cousins was proof enough that they thought I was crazy. They pointed out that I was currently single and I had never even dated a girl for a significant amount of time. They all wanted to know how was I going to not just be dating somebody, but also engaged in two years? I simply said, "I don't know, but I am ready." I proposed to Amanda less than 24 months later on February 21st, 2005. What is the moral? I didn't just want to find a girl, I was ready to find THE girl. Similarly, when I finally looked at Amanda 9 years later and said, "I am quitting sugar", I didn't want to lose weight. I wanted to fix my growing health crisis. A diet will only temporarily fix part of the problem. I needed to make a lifestyle change. There is a huge difference between the two. If you want to cut out added sugar, you have to be ready for everything that comes with it. Here are some qualifying questions you should answer yes to:

Am I ready to make a lifestyle change?

Will I be OK if weight loss isn't the first noticeable change?

Can I imagine family vacations and holidays being fun without sugar?

Am I willing to disrupt my daily routine and make new ones?

Am I willing to put the effort into finding long-term solutions and not quick fixes?

Step 2: You Have to Define What Added Sugar Means to You

I have told you how I define added sugar. I based my reasoning on both personal beliefs and sound research. Now it is time for you to do the same. Do you consider fruit juice to be added sugar? What about rice malt syrup? Did you know a girl named Sarah Wilson from Australia has a very popular website called IQuitSugar.com that is really about quitting fructose, but using rice malt syrup and stevia as approved sweeteners? Both are prohibited on my plan which happens to be very strict by comparison. This is not by accident. When you have a true sugar addiction, there has to be a zero tolerance policy. Can you imagine if an alcoholic only decided to abstain from beer and wine, but considered hard liquor OK? My point is there are a ton of different meanings to the term added sugar. You have to define what it means to you and then write it down. Post it on social media and tell your family and friends what you decided. The more people that know, the more accountable you become. To get you started, I have put together a few questions you should answer prior to your start date.

What is your take on whole fruits that are blended into a smoothie?

How do you define fruits like dates and raisins used frequently for making healthier foods taste sweeter?

How do you feel about sweeteners like stevia which come from a natural plant yet may still contribute to other sugar cravings?

What about fruit juice and fruit juice concentrates?

How about natural sweeteners like honey?

What about artificial sweeteners like aspartame?

Do you believe fructose is the only problem?

What about when sugars are used in fermentation? Such as malted barley in bread and sugar in alcohol? Do the sugars burn off and not matter?

I could go on and on with questions and you already know my take on most of these. However, I don't want to tell you how you should answer. The action plan is to go out and do some research and decide what is ultimately important to you. I find it easier to just say no to all of it, but everybody is different. Some of you reading this book are probably thinking that while you would like to reduce or eliminate your added sugar intake for health reasons, you are not a sugar addict like me. That is OK? Regardless of where you are coming from, you will see positive health benefits from reducing or eliminating added sugar from your life. The only exceptions would be if you already have a preexisting condition like diabetes or other diseases where you should absolutely consult your doctor first.

Step 3: Establish Your Own "No-Go Zones"

I talked about my own no-go zones back in the Sugar Systems chapter and now it is time for you to establish your own. These places and events will be different for everyone. For example, when my buddy at the fire station quit smoking, he also had to stop drinking Mountain Dew. Why? Because cigarettes and Mountain Dew were linked together as one social event for him. Other sodas were just fine. Eventually, he also had to stop hanging out with certain friends who still smoked. Talk about a lifestyle change. He wanted to quit smoking more than he wanted to see certain friends.

Like my fire buddy, no-go zones don't have to be physical locations. They can also include social events like holidays and other family gatherings. Now, I am in no way suggesting that you completely shut yourself in and become a sugar-free hermit. What I am suggesting is that you figure out your no-go zones early and then write down how you intend to deal with them. If it is going someplace like a gas station, that is an easy fix. You don't go inside where the problem is. However, for social events you need to fist determine why you believe the event will be a problem and then make a plan.

For example, about 1 month after I gave up added sugar, we went over to one of our client's houses for a party. I knew there was going to be a lot of food on the table, so I ate before I left the house. Since everybody at the party knew what I was doing, they went out of their way to make sure they brought other foods that I could have like basic chips and guacamole. Even with all of this prep work, I still had to come face to face with brownies and chocolate chip cookies just sitting out on the table. Had I not fully committed (Step 1), pre-determined that my answer would always be "no" (Step 2), and planned ahead for such social events (Step 3), I would have quickly broken down under the pressure and grabbed a few when nobody was looking. Instead, I was prepared and I succeeded in having a great time with our CrossFit friends without the need of sugar.

Step 4: Go Shopping

Once you have committed to the idea, defined what you will and will not eat, and determined the places and events that might cause you trouble, it is time to actually go out and buy food. Now, I already provided you with my first two weeks of grocery shopping back in Chapter 4, but you don't have to do exactly what I did. What I will suggest is make your initial plan as simple as possible. Those first few shopping trips are not the time to decide you also want to be a great chef and possibly one day publish a sugar-free recipe book. Remember, you can pursue "complicated" later. In fact, if you get this right and successfully quit added sugar, you will have the rest of your life to tinker and make amazing recipes. Right now you need the basics and the best way to do that is to stick with real foods that don't have ingredients. For example, an easy meal is a steak and baked sweet potato with some butter and cinnamon. For a vegetable, try steamed cauliflower or green beans. Round off the meal with a few toasted almonds and some fruit. Done. Now buy three times the amount you need for one meal so you don't have to cook it again a few nights later. Find about 5 other meals like this one and you will have enough to rotate through dinner and lunch for at least a few weeks without getting bored. The goal here is to get started so that you can spend your valuable time on the next step.

Step 5: Make Your Own Systems

I am a fan of systems. Not solely for helping me with my sugar addiction, but in life and business as well. You probably already have many systems in place already even if you don't call them that. For example, if you have children, you must have established some sort of system for changing diapers, feeding, washing clothes and so on. We all make systems because organization leads to cleanliness and efficiency and it is human nature to want to find the easiest route. It is no different here. The important part is that you actually develop your systems and write them down before you need them. The best time to do this? During those first few weeks while you are keeping the grocery shopping and food prep simple. Don't wait until you cannot fathom eating another steak and potato. It is too late at that point. If you are through the first 4 steps, take the time now to find easier paths in your life. I live in the suburbs so my weekly routines for shopping are going to look a lot different than somebody who lives in downtown Chicago and relies on public transport and local markets to buy their food. Where my shopping system is to always follow the same path around the store, the city-dweller might establish the same route home on certain nights of the week in order to get the fresh produce and fruit they need. Or take the police officer or firefighter who will be away from their home for multiple meals at a time. As a firefighter, I always had a cooler with me on the truck because there was no telling when the next bell would go off and how long I might be away from the station. I didn't call it a system, but that is exactly what it was. A means to make my next meal more efficient and easier to eat. Regardless of what you call it, stop now and complete this important step.

Let's review our first five steps because they are the key aspects of your action plan:

1. Commit to the lifestyle change. Go in for the right reasons.

2. Define what "no added sugar" means to you.

3. Establish your "no-go" zones and have a plan in place.

4. Go shopping for easy meals that don't stress you out.

5. Develop your own systems for making your life easier.

This brings us to the last step in the action plan.

Step 6: Test and Retest.

Remember what I told you about failing? It is going to happen. You will spend time and energy on your no-go zones, your shopping, your cooking, and your systems and not all of them will work. This is all part of the process and you need to be OK with it right now. Accept it and embrace those times as great learning opportunities. Amanda always likes to say we are all a "Study of 1". Meaning, the only plan that works for you is *your* plan. I don't have the perfect added sugar plan for you. I have suggestions and opinions based on my own life and research. I don't have the one-size fits all answer though. So you need to get out there and test and retest. Sometimes this will mean actually taking a step backwards and readdressing one of the previous steps. Perhaps you didn't define your terms well enough and now you need to make a few changes. Or maybe you fell into a trap like I did and found a few loopholes that are somehow approved on your plan and still a bad idea at the same time. It happens. I didn't mean to eat a bunch of those single serving bags of Lay's potato chips. But once I was there, I needed to stop and reevaluate what was important to me. Was it just about the fact that they didn't have added sugar? Or was I willing to admit to myself that despite the chips being "approved", they were still bad for my health and didn't fit in with my larger goal of improving my nutrition lifestyle. It is a fork in the road and nobody can tell you which is the right way to turn. Sometimes you guess correctly and sometimes you end up with potato chip crumbs on your shirt while you are driving. Life happens. Don't beat yourself up over it. Get back up and drive on.

11 GOING FORWARD

Here I am 1 year and 10 months after I began this journey.

So where do I go from here?

What is my game plan now that I am feeling great and I have been at my ideal weight for over a year and a half?

Well for starters I continue to tweak my own nutrition lifestyle and try to find ways to improve it as I mentioned in Step 6. Most recently, this came in the form of completing a Whole30 challenge for 30 days. Whole30 is an elimination plan that requires you to go without added sugar, grains, dairy, alcohol, or beans. After the 30 days, you slowly reintroduce one food at a time and wait 3 days to see if your body has an adverse reaction to it. While nothing major happened once I reintroduced grains, I can tell you I noticed feeling better without them in my life. So now I pay attention to the amount of grains I have each day and do a better job of limiting them to only one meal or not at all. I still enjoy bread immensely, but I can't deny I feel that much better without it around. My next goal is to get another set of blood work done at the 2-year mark to see if anything has changed with the reduction in grains and dairy. Beyond that, I hope to go get an MRT test done which is a blood test that looks at 150 different foods and food substances to see if I am sensitive to them or not. I am fortunate that Amanda is certified as a LEAP therapist and can help me with the results. I see it as another tool at my disposal to use for building the ultimate version of me.

The most important thing for me to do is remain vigilant. I find that when I get lazy, I miss some warning signs or have missteps. With the movement against added sugar only growing in popularity, I am certain this book will only be one of many available on the topic when it is published. While that makes me excited about getting the word out to more people, I am smart enough to know the food companies are always one step ahead of the general population. Fat free, low carb, low calorie, and gluten free are all examples of how the food industry has met public demand while simultaneously making the food we eat even worse than before. Big Soda and the sugar lobbyists will only fight the fight for so long before they realize they need to offer other solutions to appease the masses. Starbucks and other big companies have already started to pledge a reduction in sugar within x amount of time.

My prediction? "Fructose Free" will be the next big craze. Frankly, this scares the hell out of me. Because while I also believe fructose is the more dangerous simple carbohydrate, I don't trust the for-profit food industry to provide me with better alternatives. I fear a backlash over whole fruit when that isn't the problem at all. Remember what happened when they removed the fat from naturally fatty peanut butter? They added in a lot of sugar. So what can we expect when we see orange juice on the shelf at the grocery store and it is labeled "Now Fructose Free." If it does happen, I hope you will stare at the label and think, "Where did the naturally occurring fructose go?" And more importantly, "What did they replace it with and by what chemical means?"

I'm not a conspiracy theory kind of guy, but as George Santayana famously said, "Those that cannot remember the past are condemned to repeat it." I have studied the history of sugar with great detail. I have read amazing books like *Sugar Blues* and *Pure, White, and Deadly* which were published in the early 1970's and correctly predicted our sugar epidemic. I feel confident saying I understand the playbook giant corporations use to dissuade the public, or like Coke is currently doing, push an alternative agenda of eating less and moving more.

Big Tobacco used it in the 90's when they willingly sat in front of Congress and said cigarettes don't cause cancer. However, most don't realize they learned it from Big Sugar back in the 50's when dentists started connecting sugar with cavities. So it is safe to say they are using an old and effective campaign. Spend a lot of money, discredit people like myself who say they have a sugar addiction, and publish scientific documents by scientists and nutritionists on their own payroll. When all else fails, sit in front of Congress and deny, deny, deny.

Since I cannot control what the for-profit and pro-sugar industries do, I plan to continue to write and inform as many people as I can through books, public speeches, and Amanda's and my online forum, NutritionWOD.com. On the advice of our readers and subscribers, we have developed Nutrition WOD University (NWODU.com) which is a membership site where anybody can learn the proper progressions to creating an amazingly effective personalized nutrition plan. What I want most is for you to walk away from this book with is a feeling that you are not alone. Let me repeat that. If you are currently struggling with a sugar addiction, regardless of how intense, you are not alone. When I started, that is exactly how I felt. Even with all of the information on the internet, I simply felt alone and scared. Scared because I didn't know if I would fail like so many times before. Scared because I felt at 36, I was running out of opportunities to fix my health. Scared because I didn't want my own daughter to grow up and be ashamed of me one day or my wife to lose me in my 50's to diabetes or worse.

It is OK to be scared.

It is OK to be anxious.

These emotions simply mean what you are trying to accomplish is important. If nothing else, know that I have your back. I mean that. I am out there as you read this book making my own way through life, complete with my own missteps and struggles. I am testing and retesting everything. There is no one simple fix. No diet that will cure all. But I promise you this. If you give up added sugar, nothing bad will happen to you as a result of it. Nothing. You will only get healthier. You will get stronger. Your body will resist disease harder. You will have less of a chance of developing heart disease. You will lose weight. Your clothes will look different. You will feel different. You will wake up with more energy. You will be around longer for your family. You will finally wake up and remember what it is like to live. Are you ready to take the journey and change your life?

RESOURCES

I have put together some lists and information that have helped me. I have no financial ties to any products I mention aside from Trifecta Nutrition which pays me a small percentage when people sign up for their meal delivery service. You can be assured though that I not only use their meals to help me stay on track, but that any partnership made was done after Amanda and I thoroughly vetted the company for high standards. Aside from product suggestions, you will find the books I read, documentaries I watched, Facebook pages I like, websites I visit, podcasts I listen to in the car, apps I use daily on my phone, and online services I love. Aside from Fed Up which was a bigger catalyst for my change, all of these resources have had an impact on my life and have in some way shaped who I am and what I believe today. As I grow and learn more, my opinions may change and I think that is a great thing. I hope to write the follow up to this book in a few years to tell you all what I have been doing and how I have continued to evolve.

Books

Pure, White, and Deadly by John Yudkin

This book was first published in 1972. The scary part is when you read it you would swear it was written last year. Here is a quote from the book. "I believe that the best diet for the human species is one made up as far as possible of the foods that were available in our hunting and food gathering days." Thought the Paleo Diet was a relatively new idea? Not so much. John was talking about it 40 years ago and essentially saying we should all get back to eating real foods. I couldn't agree more and I highly recommend this landmark book.

Sugar Blues by William Dufty

Published in 1975, William Dufty was inspired by his famous wife Gloria Swanson who lived a sugar-free lifestyle. What makes this book different is that it is a history book at heart. Dufty weaves the story of sugar into the history of civilization and makes an interesting case for sugar being at the center of it all.

It Starts With Food by Melissa and Dallas Hartwig

This is the book that launched the successful Whole30 Challenge. Regardless of whether you want to take the 30 day challenge or not, I highly recommend this easy to read book.

Soda Politics by Marion Nestle

Here is a more recent book about Big Soda and what can be accomplished with billions in marketing with nothing more than flavored sugar water. If you weren't aware of how big the sugar industry is and how important it is to protect for these large companies, you will after reading this book.

Always Hungry? by David Ludwig

Another recent book that I enjoyed. Dr Ludwig has been studying sugar and obesity for decades and this is his take on how to fix it through diet.

In Defense of Food - Michael Pollan

It is hard to believe this book is 8 years old because we refer back to it all of the time. He has a famous prescription that says, "Eat food. Not too much. Mostly plants." You can't say it any more succinct. It is a famous book for good reason and definitely worth your time to read.

That Sugar Book - Damon Gameau

This is the companion book to the documentary That Sugar Film. Both the book and the film are exceptional and I highly recommend reading and watching.

Facebook Pages

Fooducate - Not all of their posts are on point with what I believe, but I like most of them and often share them on Nutrition WOD's page.

Tastemade - They make short videos of food recipes look so enticing. Not exactly a sugar-free page, but there are plenty of healthy recipes on their website and YouTube page.

Whole30 Recipes - A great resource

Whole30 - Always something valuable being shared on their page.

Institute for Responsible Nutrition - A non-profit started in part by Robert Lustig.

Stupid Easy Paleo - Steph Gaurdreau has been an ambassador of the Paleo lifestyle for several years and I like that she practices what she preaches.

Dr. Joseph Mercola - Sometimes the posts are a bit out there, but more than not, there is some great information about eating healthy and surrounding yourself with healthy products. I can get behind that idea.

That Sugar Film - Despite the documentary coming out last year, this page continues to be active and director Damon Gameau is proving to be a voice for change.

Websites

ResponsibleFoods.org - This is the website for Institute for Responsible Nutrition - The main board member is Robert Lustig, but there are a lot of other qualified contributors.

IQuitSugar.com - This is the companion website to Australian author Sarah Wilson. My only complaint about this otherwise helpful site is when Sarah says she quit sugar, she means she quit fructose, but not rice malt syrup and stevia. Both of these are prohibited in my book if you want to say you quit added sugar. To Sarah's credit, she explains her reasons in full on her site and admits "I Quit Sugar" is a catchier title than "I Quit Fructose."

DrHyman.com - This is the site for Dr. Mark Hyman who has been around for years touting the benefits of eating real food and avoiding added sugar. He is a charismatic guy who is the face of a much larger website. I would imagine he has a team of people working on new content for his site and I generally find the information fact-based and useful.

Documentaries

Fed Up - This is the documentary that started my final drive toward improving my health and life. I watched it in the theaters with Amanda and it began to click that my problem wasn't my ability to count calories or work out hard enough. My problem was I had an addiction to sugar and I didn't know it. My outlook changed after this documentary for me. I owe a lot to Katie Couric and filmmaker Stephanie Soechtig.

Forks Over Knives - An interesting film about how eating a plant based diet over a predominantly animal based one can help control or even eliminate diseases.

In Defense of Food - Michael Pollan's documentary that accompanies the book by the same title. I like it because it is not an expert touting research as much as it is a common man taking a step back and saying, "This doesn't make sense. Maybe we are looking at this the wrong way." Recently, he also released a mini documentary series on Netflix called *Cooked* that is also interesting.

That Sugar Film - Damon Gameau took a Supersize Me type approach to added sugar by only eating foods that were thought to be healthy, yet filled with sugar. It is an eye-opening film because it show how even those with the best of intentions, can mistakenly eat tons of added sugar while believing they are making healthier choices.

Food, Inc. - You won't be able to say you didn't know after watching this revealing film about the state of our food industry. Robert Kenner, the filmmaker, might convince you to change your ways.

Mobile Apps

Fooducate - I have tried and tested many apps over the years. This is my favorite.

Healthy Out - A quick reference guide to eating out and making healthier decisions. It comes in handy when you are on the run.

In R Food - Similar to Fooducate and Healthy Out, In R Food has a great ingredient look up. Wondering what brown rice syrup is? Type it in and get some quick answers while standing in the grocery store.

My app - As in this doesn't exist yet, but I want it to. I basically want to be able to walk into my local grocery store (Publix or Whole Foods) and have an app that basically gives me an augmented reality overlay of the store as I walk in. So if I only want to buy products without added sugar, it will highlight exactly where to look as I walk down the aisles or point my phone at a wall full of choices. I don't have a ton of time to pull each product off the shelf and read the back of it. So if an app could color code what I am looking at through my phone, I could easily determine anything that is green is a possible winner. Now instead of 20 choices, I have 2 or 3 and that not only helps me save time, but make better choices on the fly. Plus, when I return for a follow up visit, the app would know what I bought last time and help me devise the quickest route to grab it and go. Oh, and I want the coupons to be on there too. Is that too much to ask?

Podcasts

BulletProof Radio - Dave Asprey This is the guy who made bulletproof coffee a thing. I find the podcast is always interesting and he is knowledgeable.

Barbell Shrugged - While the crew has changed a bit, I still enjoy this podcast because it is just a bunch of guys talking about CrossFit, diet, and working out. It is more of a lifestyle podcast over a nutrition one, but I always find some nugget to take with me.

Nutrition WOD's Daily Bites - What can I say? I like listening to myself on the radio in my car. It is the closest I will ever get to the real thing and it is a cool feeling thinking there might be somebody in their car who is listening to me and getting their own nugget.

Online Services

WellnessFx - I am a fan of owning my own medical records. Call me crazy, but I don't like having to call my PCP to get a copy of my stuff. Now I don't have to. All of the blood work I had done over the past two years has been done through WellnessFx. I pay online, I give a blood sample, and in a few days I get a great report back that tells me everything I need to know in one online format.

Food and Food Services

Epic Bar - I mentioned them in the book. Their animal protein bars are great and make for a quick snack on the run. I prefer them cold out of the fridge, but they can sit on a shelf too. epicbar.com

Core - Love these guys. They run a non-profit and are the sort of people you wish lived closer so you could go hang out with them and learn something new. corefoods.com

Trifecta Nutrition - The only company I have a financial tie to on this list. We found their food online. Amanda was impressed with their level of dedication to meal prep. We tried some food out. We loved it. We kept buying it. THEN we spoke to the owners about bringing it to more people. What can I say? I would promote them for free. But it is nice to know Trifecta values the people we bring to them. NutritionWOD.com/trifecta

Bare Snacks - Cinnamon Banana Chips - I wish I had stock in this company. I eat these chips all of the time and I love them. Two ingredients: Bananas and Cinnamon. They are crunchy and they satisfy any cravings I might have for other chips. baresnacks.com

Wildway - A great find by Amanda on a trip to D.C. in 2015. They make these cool to-go cups that remind me of ramen noodles. Unlike the sodium filled ramen, this is a mix of nuts and seeds and I love mixing it with some coconut milk, frozen cherries, and a fresh cut banana in the morning. Wildwayoflife.com.

ABOUT THE AUTHOR

Brian Maucere has over 20 years and 10,000 hours of coaching experience. With his wife Amanda, who is a dietitian, they ran a successful CrossFit gym for 5 years before deciding to sell it so they could focus on helping people with their nutrition goals. They took over NutritionWOD.com and now help thousands of people around the world. In 2014, Brian decided to quit all added sugar after realizing his own health was suffering. Using his background as a coach and mentor, Brian began helping others with their own sugar addictions. Now almost 2 years after quitting, Brian is releasing his first book on how he did it and the tools others can use to do the same. Brian and Amanda have one daughter, Sofia, who was Brian's inspiration to both quit added sugar and write this book.